SOTHIS PRESS

Sothis Press aims to completely reimagine the public domain book with an emphasis on universal access to captivatingly designed print editions. We believe that technology will enable every single book ever published to be perpetually accessible in beautiful print form. Sothis is beauty in ubiquity.

www.sothis.press
1 Waterhouse Square, London, ECIN 2ST

Cicuta, or Water Hemlock

C. Dwight Marsh

SOTHIS PRESS

ISBN 978-1-0365-1129-6

Cicuta, or Water Hemlock
is in the public domain.

BULLETIN OF THE U.S. DEPARTMENT OF AGRICULTURE

No. 69

Contribution from the Bureau of Plant Industry, Wm. A. Taylor, Chief, and the Bureau of Animal Industry, A. D. Melvin, Chief.
March 28, 1914.

(PROFESSIONAL PAPER.)

CICUTA, OR WATER HEMLOCK.

By C. Dwight Marsh and A. B. Clawson, *Physiologists, Drug-Plant and Poisonous-Plant Investigations, Bureau of Plant Industry*, and Hadleigh Marsh, *Veterinary Inspector, Bureau of Animal Industry*.

INTRODUCTION.

HISTORICAL SUMMARY.

Among poisonous plants the genus Cicuta is of especial interest, as it is probably the most violently toxic of all the plants growing in temperate regions. Since the middle of the sixteenth century the genus has been definitely known, and the symptoms produced by it have been accurately described many times. Before that time, if recognized at all, it was not distinguished from Conium. The term Cicuta occurs frequently in Latin literature, but without any doubt was used as the equivalent of the Greek *Κωνειον*. Whether the hemlock used by the Greeks and Romans for the punishment of criminals and for suicidal purposes was an extract from a single plant or a compound extract of several plants, as thought by some, may never be known, but in any case it is evident that plants of the genus Cicuta as recognized to-day were not used. The symptoms produced by the hemlock are described in detail by Plato in connection with the death of Socrates and are very different from those produced by Cicuta. There seems to be little doubt that Conium was the principal constituent of the hemlock and perhaps the only substance used.

Albert Regel, 1876–77,[1] has gone into great detail in discussing the history of the "hemlock" and "water hemlock," with copious quotations from ancient authors. Inasmuch as Cicuta is not found in any abundance in Greece and Italy, it may, perhaps, fairly be questioned whether the Greeks and Romans had any knowledge of the

[1] For complete titles of works cited in this bulletin, see list on pages 24 to 27.

NOTE.—This bulletin describes water hemlock and its toxic effect upon animal life when taken into the system; it points out the distinction between it and other umbelliferous plants, particularly conium, with which it is most likely to be confounded. As the toxic principle is largely confined to the rootstock, the tops and seeds if they become mixed with hay are not a source of danger. The subject is of general interest, as cicuta is found in nearly all parts of the United States.

plant. To Konrad Gesner is generally given the credit of first clearly distinguishing Cicuta from Conium. In 1541, in his Historia Plantarum, he speaks of it as Sium, but later he calls it *Cicuta aquatica.* In his edition of Dioscorides, 1543, he says "Recentiores faciunt duo genera, aquaticae frigentis naturae, terrestris calide: verum quonam nullum idoneum praeferunt autorem, vereor ne, ut feresolent, hallucinentur." By the first he probably means Cicuta, and by the second, Conium. In 1561, in "Horti Germaniae," f. 253, he says "*Cicuta aquatica,* herba venenosa, Bartzenkraut Saxonibus, G. Circa paludes & in paludum marginibus sponte oritur, ut ad lacum Felium agri Tigurini plantare si quis velit, in aqua aut loco palustri pangatur oportet."

In 1679 was published "Cicutae Aquaticae Historia et Noxae," by J. J. Wepfer. This book of 336 pages is a rather elaborate work, based on a case of poisoning in which two boys and six girls were involved. In the first nine chapters, comprising about one-half the book, the plant is described and a detailed account of the cases of poisoning given; there is a discussion of the symptoms, of the physiology and pharmacology of the cases, and details of the autopsies are given. In the tenth chapter is an account of some experimental work. In the chapters from the eleventh to the twenty-first, inclusive, other poisons are taken up and discussed. The twenty-second chapter is concerned with the uses of Cicuta, and the twenty-third and last with remedial measures in cases of poisoning. While written in a diffuse style, with much extraneous matter and containing many errors, it is on the whole a very remarkable work. When treating of facts Wepfer's statements are clear-cut and accurate. His description of the symptoms of the poisoned children is not only one of the best accounts of the symptoms of Cicuta poisoning ever written, but is handled in a graphic style that could hardly be excelled. (See pp. 17–18.)

In 1687 Wepfer published a short paper giving details in regard to four cases of poisoning, one of them being fatal. While Gesner was the first to distinguish what is now known as Cicuta in his *Cicuta aquatica,* Wepfer was the first to set forth clearly the peculiar poisonous properties of Cicuta.

Wepfer attempts to give the synonomy of preceding authors; for example, he gives—

Oenanthe cicutae facie succo viroso crocante Lobel, 1570, p. 326.
Cicutaria palustris tenuifolia Bauhin, 1623. Lib. IV, Sec. V, p. 161.
Cicuta aquatica Gesneri Bauhin, 1651. Lib. XXVII, p. 175.

In regard to these and other identifications, it may be said that the plant descriptions of that time were not complete enough to make identification certain from morphological characters. The habits of these two genera, Conium and Cicuta, however, sometimes show pretty clearly which is meant. Conium grows in fairly dry ground in the neighborhood of towns, while Cicuta grows in wet places. So when Ray speaks of *Cicutaria palustris*, 1704, Lib. VIII, p. 257, we can be reasonably certain that he means Cicuta. If the symptoms of poisoning are given, as in Wepfer's work, the identity of the plant is without question.

During the seventeenth century Cicuta was mentioned by other authors, but little was written of it as a poisonous plant.

In 1723 Helds, Weinmann, and Goritz described a case of three students near Regensburg who ate the root of *Cicuta virosa* with resulting illness and two fatalities. There are three independent accounts, one by each of the writers mentioned, and the symptoms and autopsy findings are described in some detail. Weinmann tells of the death of seven persons near Nuremberg. Goritz grew the plant and gives a description of it.

The next account of importance was by Schwencke in 1756. The original paper was in Dutch, but a German translation by Müller was published in 1776. After a description of the plant he gives the details of the poisoning of four children near the village of Overschie. They were left to themselves in their home, and the mother on her return found them scattered about the floor "struggling with death." Three of the four died. Autopsies were made on two, and Schwencke gives the details of the autopsies and discusses the symptoms fully.

Up to the nineteenth century there were many other references to Cicuta, some of which gave some little information in regard to its poisonous properties, but the foregoing account includes the more important papers. All of these accounts were concerned with the European species, *Cicuta virosa.*

During the nineteenth century a large number of cases of poisoning by *Cicuta virosa* were reported, the greater number being in Germany. These reports bear a close resemblance to each other. Most of the cases were of children, and the descriptions of symptoms differ but little, except that in some cases greater detail is given. Much of this literature will be referred to in the further discussion of the subject.

Apparently the first mention of Cicuta as a poisonous plant in America was by Schwencke, who speaks of it as the Virginian "Wasser Schierling." Schoepf, in his Materia Medica Americana, 1787, makes the following statement: "Ob affinitatem genericam cum Cicuta virosa partim, suspecta esse deberet; id quod testimonium Schwenkii, de Cicuta aquatica, p. 28, confirmat, qui hanc plantam Cephalalgiam et vertiginem causare dicit."

In this connection it should perhaps be noted that the so-called *Cicuta venenosa* described in connection with a case of poisoning by Greenway, 1793, was not Cicuta. In the Kew index this name is given as a synonym of *Angelica hirsuta, A. villosa.* The symptoms described do not at all correspond to those produced by Cicuta.

Stockbridge, 1814, tells of the poisoning of three boys, with one fatality, giving details of the symptoms and treatment. He tells also of another case of a boy 6 or 7 years old who died after violent convulsive fits "and the most awful and exquisite sufferings I ever witnessed."

Ely and Muhlenberg, 1815, tell of a similar case of three boys, two of whom died. Bigelow, 1817, describes the plant, giving a general statement in regard to its poisonous properties, and refers to the cases mentioned by Stockbridge and Ely.

Hazeltine, 1818, tells of the "fatal effects of a poisonous root." He did not identify the plant, but his account of the symptoms makes it certain that it was *Cicuta maculata.*

During the nineteenth century a considerable literature in regard to poisoning by Cicuta in North America grew up, a large part of it relating to losses of live stock, although there have been very many recorded cases of the poisoning of human beings, and it is known that many cases, perhaps the larger number, have not been published. Most of these accounts are more or less fragmentary in character, and it is not considered necessary to give a synopsis of them.

THE GENUS CICUTA.

The following description of the genus Cicuta is compiled from the last edition of Gray's Manual: [1]

> A perennial umbellifer growing from a rootstock, with pinnately compound leaves and serrate leaflets. Involucre usually none, involucels of several slender bractlets, flowers white. Fruit ovoid to nearly orbicular, glabrous, with strong, flattish, corky ribs, the lateral largest; oil tubes conspicuous, solitary; stylopodium depressed; seed nearly terete.

The genus is distributed in the northern continents. A large number of species have been described, most of which are so closely related to each other that in many cases the validity of the species has been questioned. The common species of the eastern United States is *maculata,* which has been, by some, considered as not specifically distinct from the European *virosa.*

Probably all species are equally poisonous, and in popular parlance no distinction of species is made.

DISTINCTION BETWEEN CICUTA AND CONIUM.

From the standpoint of a poisonous plant Cicuta is more likely to be confounded with Conium than with any other umbelliferous plant.

---

[1] Seventh edition, p. 614.

For comparison with the diagnosis of Cicuta there follows a diagnosis of Conium compiled from Gray's Manual:[1]

A biennial umbellifer with spotted stems, large decompound leaves with lanceolate pinnatifid leaflets. Involucre and involucels of narrow bracts, flowers white. Fruit ovate, flattened at the sides, glabrous, with prominent wavy ribs; oil tubes none, but a layer of secreting cells next the seed, the face of which is deeply and narrowly concave.

Leaves and flowers of water hemlock (*Cicuta vagans*) are shown in Plate I, while a young plant of the same species is illustrated in Plate II. For comparison, a branch of *Conium maculatum* is shown in Plate III.

It will be seen that Cicuta and Conium are clearly distinguished morphologically by the leaves and fruit and by the presence of an involucre in Conium and its absence in Cicuta. These characteristics, however, are hardly sufficient to enable one unskilled in botany to make the distinction readily.

A peculiarity of the rootstock which is not mentioned by the systematic botanists makes it comparatively easy to distinguish Cicuta from any other umbellifer that is likely to be found in the same locality. If the rootstock is cut longitudinally there will be seen, more or less clearly, a number of transverse chambers, as shown in Plate II.

These chambers are not as distinct in the spring as later in the season, but they can always be recognized. This peculiarity of the root was noted in Flora Danica in 1765, a figure showing the chambers. They were mentioned by Trumel, 1838, and Maly, 1844, and have been figured by a number of more recent authors. It should be noted, too, that while Conium grows in fields and waste places, Cicuta grows in wet places, like swamps and along irrigating ditches, the old specific name *aquatica* being a particularly appropriate one.

POPULAR NAMES.

Among English-speaking people the Cicuta is most commonly known as "water hemlock" or "cowbane." Other names are "parsnip" (or "wild parsnip"), "snakeroot," "spotted hemlock," "spotted parsley," "snakeweed," "beaver poison," "musquash root," and "muskrat weed."

In New Mexico it has been known as "pecos." According to Muhlenberg, an Indian name was "utcum."

Among the Germans it is known as "Wasserschierling," sometimes as "giftiger Schierling." "Schierling" seems to be more commonly applied to Conium, although apparently this distinction between "Wasserschierling" and "Schierling" is not always made. It is also known as "Wüterich," "giftiger Wüterich," "Parzenkraut," "Tollkraut," and "Tollrube."

---

[1] Seventh edition, p. 613.

By the French it is known as "Ciguë vireuse," "Ciguë tachetée" being applied to Conium.

SPECIES OF CICUTA REPORTED AS POISONOUS.

The following species of Cicuta have been reported as poisonous: *C. maculata, bulbifera, vagans, bolanderi, occidentalis, californica, curtisii, douglasii, purpurea, tenuifolia,* and *virosa*. In some cases this belief is supported by strong experimental evidence. This evidence is especially strong in regard to *maculata, vagans, occidentalis, californica,* and *virosa*. There is every reason to believe that all species of Cicuta are poisonous, and possibly all equally so.

LOCALITIES WHERE CICUTA POISONING HAS OCCURRED.

The number of reported cases of poisoning by Cicuta in Europe is very large, by far the greater number having occurred in Germany.

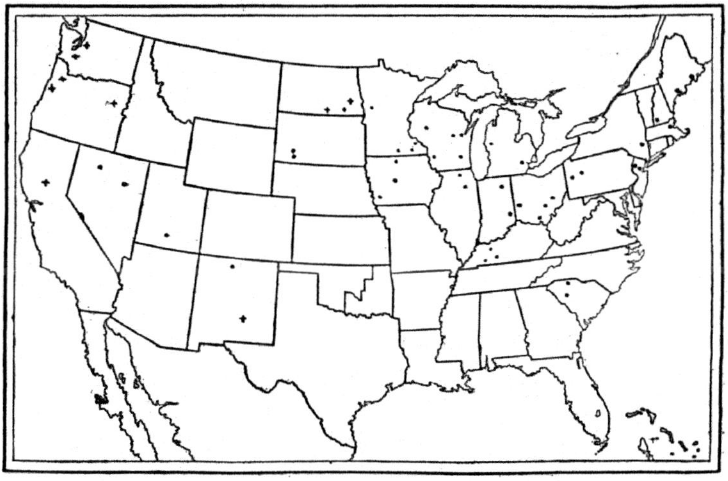

FIG. 1.—Map of the United States, showing the distribution of recorded cases of poisoning by Cicuta. Dots indicate the locations of poisoning of human beings, while crosses show the locations of cattle poisoning.

In figure 1 the recorded cases of poisoning in the United States have been plotted, dots indicating the places where members of the human family have been poisoned, while crosses show the localities of cattle poisoning. This chart has been compiled from publications and from definite records in the Office of Poisonous Plants of the United States Department of Agriculture. The first published account was by Stockbridge, 1814. Figure 1 by no means represents the entire number of cases. The compilation of this chart brought out in a surprising manner how imperfectly such cases have been put on record. For example, there seems to be no definite record of poisoning in Montana. Yet in the year 1900 alone, according to Chesnut and Wilcox, there were five cases of poisoning of human beings in the State, resulting in four fatalities, and a loss of 30 head of cattle and 80 sheep. These could not be plotted, as no definite localities were given. The writers of this bulletin have been informed of many losses of cattle in Colorado, but no accounts were sufficiently definite to admit of plotting.

In regard to sheep, we have a definite local record of only one case of poisoning, at Klamath Falls, Oreg. Yet the yearly losses are heavy. Figure 1, then, must not be considered as giving more than a very incomplete record.

The greater number of cases recorded in the East as compared with the West is partly due to the greater density of population and partly to the special interest taken in the subject in some localities. The number of locations in Wisconsin is largely due to the interest which Prof. Power took in verifying reported cases in that State.

LOSSES OF LIVE STOCK FROM CICUTA POISONING IN THE UNITED STATES.

There are no data from which we can make a reliable estimate of the stock losses from Cicuta poisoning. One man in Oregon, presumably estimating the loss in his immediate neighborhood, makes it 10 per cent. Slade, 1903, estimates a loss of a hundred head of cattle a year in Oregon.

Chesnut and Wilcox, 1901, say that in 1900 in Montana 30 head of cattle and 80 head of sheep were lost. Probably the losses in the aggregate are very small. Individual owners of stock have occasionally lost rather heavily, but the total loss does not compare at all with the deaths from other poisonous plants, such plants, for example, as the locos and larkspurs.

USES OF CICUTA.

Most plant substances with positive, evident characteristics have been assumed to have properties useful in medicine. As would be supposed, Cicuta, with its violent toxic character, has attracted attention and has been used for a great variety of diseases. Wepfer, 1679, Chapter XXII, discusses its uses in some detail, but most, if not all, that he says refers to Conium rather than Cicuta.

Gadd, 1774, says that the Finns drive crickets from their homes with Cicuta. It may be questioned, however, whether this is anything more than a story that he had heard.

In later times Cicuta has been used in medicine to a limited extent. Rafinesque, 1828, p. 110, says:

> A few grains have been given in schirrose and scrofulous tumors and ulcers, with equal advantage, but a larger dose produces nausea and vomiting; the doses should be very small, often repeated, and gradually increased. It has been used as a gargle for sore throat, but safer substances ought to be preferred.

In Siberia the crushed nut is used for syphilitic symptoms, and in Norway for gout, while the seeds have been used as a diuretic.[1]

In the nineteenth edition of Wood and Bache's Dispensatory of the United States, p. 1449, are the following statements: "At present the plant (*Cicuta virosa*) is never used internally, and rarely externally as an anodyne poultice in local pains."

"*Cicuta* (*maculata*) has been highly lauded as a specific in nervous and sick headache, but is rarely, if ever, used." (Stearns, 1858, p. 253.)

Dragendorff, 1898, p. 487, states that in Oregon Cicuta is used as an arrow poison.

Cicuta has sometimes been used for committing suicide, although it is probable that the statement which is made by some writers to the effect that it was kept by the people of Marseilles for this purpose is inaccurate, as it is more likely that Conium was used.

Rafinesque, 1828, page 110, says "The Indians when tired of life are said to poison themselves with the roots of this plant."

Caillard, 1829, tells of a laborer who purchased and ate the root for suicidal purposes, but recovered after being given an emetic.

Trojanowsky, 1874, relates how a laborer, after a drunken spree and a domestic quarrel, left home and was the next day found dead, the cause of death being Cicuta. The evidence was considered sufficient to prove that he ate the root of *Cicuta virosa* with the deliberate purpose of committing suicide.

Trojanowsky refers also to another case, the "Kobeilla'sche Process," but it has been impossible to verify this, as the reference in Trojanowsky's paper is evidently wrong.

Přibram, 1900, tells of an interesting case. A woman having suffered considerable domestic infelicity, on her way to arrange for a divorce called on a fortune teller to find out whether she would succeed in the separation. The fortune teller told her that the separation was unnecessary, as her husband would not live more than one year and advised her to measure the shadow of her husband with a stick, throw the stick upon a stream, saying "I lay down not this stick but thy life, and as the stick becomes broken in its passage, so shall thy life be cut off." Upon the woman replying that she did not wish her husband to die, the fortune teller went to a swamp and gathered three roots, calling them "neapte de boalta," and told her to make a mash of two of these roots, two potatoes, some corn meal, sheep cheese, and onions, and bake a cake of it for her husband to eat. After eating this root, her husband would go about for three months in a stunned condition and would not abuse her or compel her to live with him. If her husband after eating the cake should become ill, the fortune teller would give her tea, so that he should not die.

---

[1] Brandt, Phoebus, and Ratzeburg, 1838, p. 111.

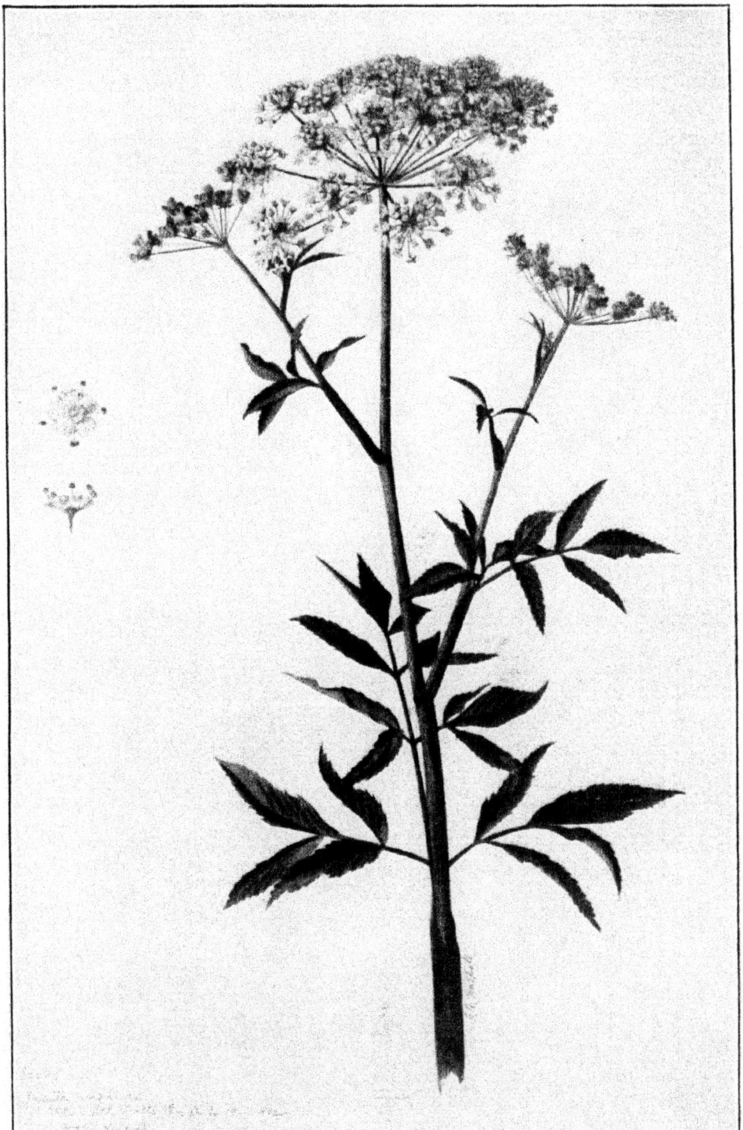

CICUTA VAGANS, SHOWING LEAVES AND FLOWERS.

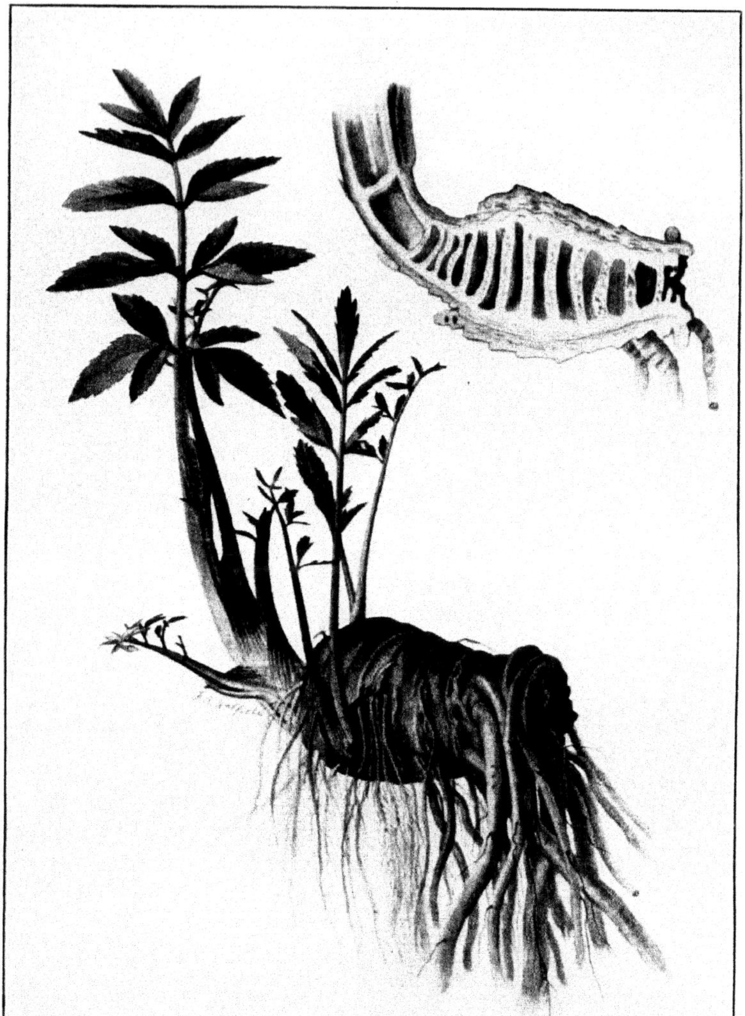

A YOUNG PLANT OF CICUTA VAGANS, SHOWING THE FORM OF THE ROOTSTOCK.

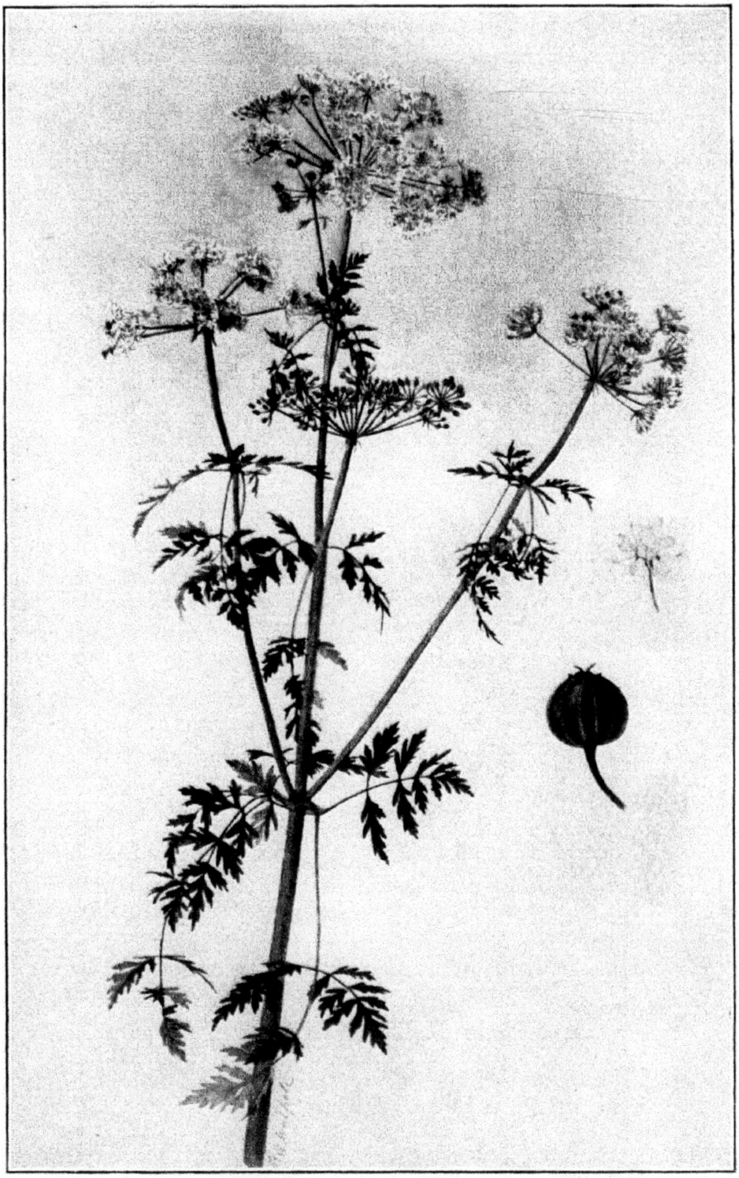

CONIUM MACULATUM, SHOWING LEAVES, FLOWERS, AND FRUITS.

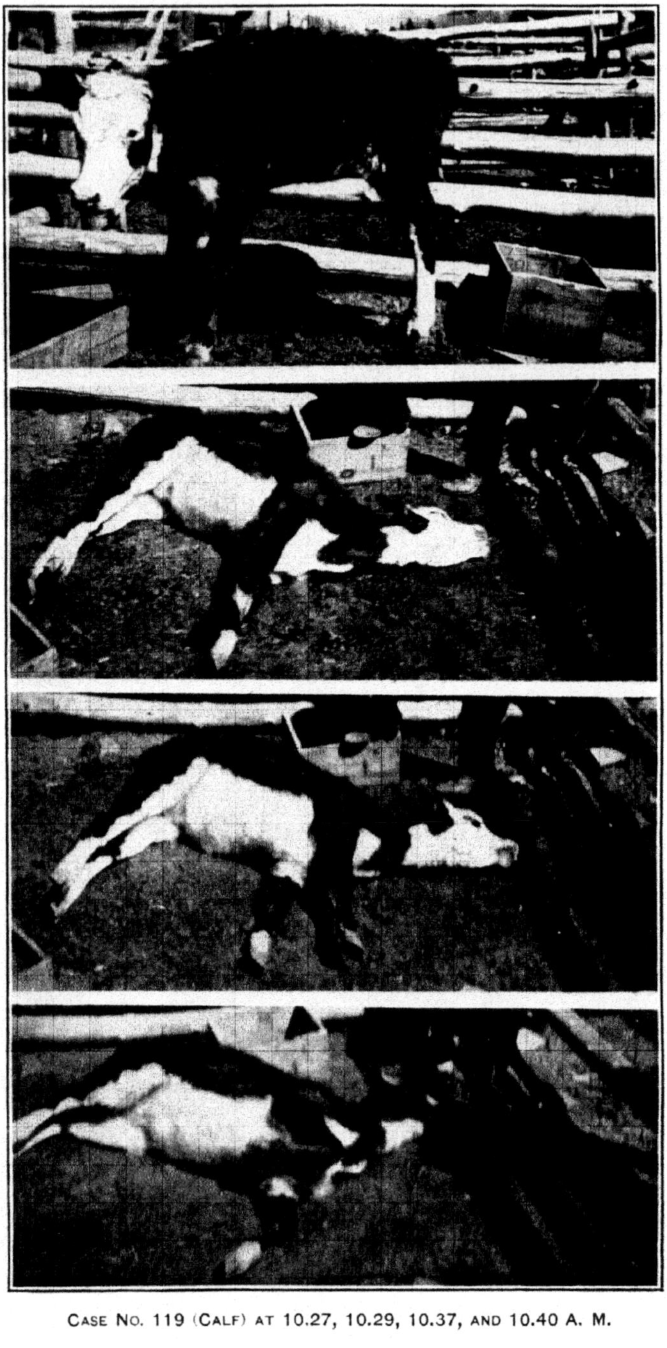

CASE NO. 119 (CALF) AT 10.27, 10.29, 10.37, AND 10.40 A. M.

The woman followed these directions, using one root instead of two. An hour later her husband complained of pain and was nauseated, afterwards falling senseless. Apparently he did not entirely lose consciousness, for he was helped into the home and sat down, but soon fell unconscious and shortly afterwards died, his death occurring about two hours after eating the cake.

It was shown by examination that the root furnished by the fortune teller was that of *Cicuta virosa*.

THE POISONOUS PRINCIPLE OF CICUTA.

When the rootstock of Cicuta is cut open, drops of an aromatic oil are noted, which give the root its peculiar odor, and this oil is popularly thought to be the poisonous substance. The poisonous principle, however, is not in the oil but in a resin, and has been separated under the name of cicutoxin and especially studied by Boehm, 1875-76, Wikzemski, 1875, and Pohl, 1894. It has properties similar to picrotoxin and with these two are commonly grouped coriamyrtin, œnanthotoxin, and santonin.

Kunkel, 1901, p. 934, describes this poisonous principle as a clear brown, sticky resin with an acid reaction, which does not harden when dried. It is soluble in ether, alcohol, chloroform, and dilute alkalis, and is precipitated from alkaline solutions by acids. It is slightly soluble in cold water and more readily in hot water.

Wikzemski, 1875, gives in detail the results of subcutaneous injections of the poison in frogs. His conclusions are as follows:

(1) The poisonous principle of *Cicuta virosa* produces in frogs clonic-tonic convulsions of the whole body and in doses of 4 to 6 milligrams of the ether extract kills with paralysis.

(2) The effect of the poison limits itself to the central nervous system. The activity of the heart and organs of respiration is influenced in a secondary way.

(3) The principal effect of the Cicuta poison is upon the "convulsion center" at the end of the medulla oblongata. The upper part of the brain is not affected, while the terminal paralysis of the spinal cord apparently results from the complete exhaustion following the convulsions.

EXPERIMENTAL WORK.

EXPERIMENTS IN COLORADO.

Cicuta occidentalis grew in considerable abundance along the ditches in the irrigated land of Ohio Creek Valley, Colo., at the head of which the Mount Carbon Station was located. The ranchers recognize it as a poisonous plant and some of them make a business of cutting it out. It is never, however, entirely destroyed, and sometimes large quantities of it are cut with the hay.

The experimental work had three objects in view:

(1) To determine whether the plant was poisonous in summer and early fall.

(2) To settle definitely the question of the danger to live stock from eating hay containing Cicuta.

(3) To obtain material for verifying and amplifying the description of symptoms and the effects of Cicuta poisoning.

This work was carried on in the summers of 1910 and 1911.

FEEDING CICUTA TO SHEEP IN 1910.

In Table I is given a summarized account of the sheep-feeding experiments of 1910. The details of the cases follow. An attempt was made to feed two other sheep, but neither could be induced to eat the material.

TABLE I.—*Summary of feeding experiments with Cicuta occidentalis, 1910. (Sheep.)*

Animal.	Weight.	Amount fed.	Period of feeding.	Part of plant fed.
	Pounds.	*Pounds.*		
No. 108	100	51.5	Aug. 14 to 23	Roots, stems, leaves, and seeds.
No. 104	91	41	Aug. 26 to Sept. 9	Roots.
No. 125	100	91	Aug. 26 to Sept. 11	Stems, leaves and seed.
No. 102	93	2.5	Sept. 15 to 16	Roots.
No. 101	96	(Very little.)	Sept. 15 to 21	Do.
No. 115	48	(Very little.)	Sept. 17 to 21	Do.

Animal.	Period of sickness (until able to stand).	Remedy used.	Result.	Ratio of plant fed to weight of animal.	Amount fed to 100 pounds of weight of animal.	Location from which plant fed was obtained.
					Pounds.	
No. 108	Short attack; 35 minutes.	Potassium permanganate.	Recovery.	1: 1.9	51.5	Sellinger.
No. 104	About 1 minute; 1 to 2 minutes; 23 minutes	None	do	1: 2.3	45	Allison.
No. 125		do	Not sick	1: 1.1	91	Do.
No. 102		do	Death	1:37.2	2.7	Do.
No. 101		do	Not sick			Do.
No. 115		do	do			Do.

CASE No. 108.

Case No. 108, a wether weighing 100 pounds, was taken out of the pasture on the night of August 12 for feeding with Cicuta. The feeding was commenced at 11.30 a. m. on August 14, when he was given ground tubers of *Cicuta occidentalis.* During the day he ate very little except what he got accidentally in picking out oats that had been thrown upon the ground material. On the morning of August 15 he was given an additional quantity of Cicuta roots, this being mixed with hay with the feed that had remained from the preceding day. Apparently very little of this was eaten except what was obtained accidentally in connection with taking the hay, but by the night of August 16 he had eaten a considerable amount of roots. On August 17 he was fed stems and tops of Cicuta, the plant being in seed. This was entirely eaten up with what remained of the Cicuta roots by the night of August 17. On the morning of August 18 more of the ground roots was fed with cut hay and it was all eaten. Because of lack of material he was not fed on August 19. On August 20 and 21 he was fed stems, leaves, and seeds. Up to this time no effects had been noticed from the feeding.

On the morning of August 22 he was again given ground Cicuta roots in cut hay, receiving at this time 2 pounds. At 12.30 noon, the animal was found down and apparently unable to get up when disturbed, but when raised to his feet was able to stand. He frothed a little at the mouth. About 15 minutes later he appeared to be all right and ran about the corral actively. No further symptoms were noticed on this day.

On the morning of August 23, at 8.30 a. m., this sheep was given 5 pounds of ground Cicuta roots in cut hay. At 6.30 p. m. he was found lying down on his side with legs extended and with head raised and turned to one side. His eyes were turned down, showing the white above the iris. His breathing was rapid and noisy, groans accompanying the expirations. When raised on his legs he stood for a minute with hind legs braced apart and stretched out behind, then trembled violently and fell, acting as if he were choking. Potassium permanganate and aluminium sulphate were administered in a drench, although it was difficult to make him swallow. He kept his mouth closed tight and ground his teeth together. At 6.45 his pulse was 176. At 7 his respiration was 62, apparently growing slower. At 7.05 he got upon his feet with assistance and stood with his legs braced apart. His pulse was 180, full and strong. At 7.08 his respiration was 46 and the groaning had ceased. At 7.15 the pulse was 168 and respiration 26. At 7.20 his pulse was 168. Some of this time he remained on his feet, gradually growing stronger, and at 8.30 had walked a few steps. At that time he was stupid and weak. When he walked he staggered and dragged his hind feet. His pulse was 84, respiration 20.

On the morning of August 24, while somewhat weak and uncertain on his feet, he appeared fairly well and was turned into the pasture, showing no further symptoms. His weight at that time was 91 pounds, showing that in the course of the experiment he had lost 9 pounds. On the last day of the feeding, August 23, of the 5 pounds of Cicuta roots he had eaten about 3½ pounds.

The impression from the experiment was that the stems, leaves, and seeds had been fed without effect and that the poisoning was directly the result of feeding the roots on August 23.

Case No. 104.

Case No. 104 was brought in from the pasture for Cicuta feeding on August 24. This wether weighed 91 pounds at 6 p. m. on August 25. Feeding was commenced at 9.50 a. m., August 26, when he was given 2½ pounds of ground Cicuta roots mixed with a pound of cut hay. He did not eat readily, but during the day disposed of perhaps two-thirds of the amount fed in the morning.

On August 27 part of the feed remaining was removed and more was supplied in cut hay. Feeding was carried on in this manner through August 28, 29, 30, and 31. During the day of August 31 he had eaten all the Cicuta supplied and was given some additional hay.

On September 1, the supply of Cicuta being exhausted, he was fed hay. The feeding of the ground roots was resumed on September 2 and continued until the morning of September 8 before any results were noted.

At a little after 10 a. m., September 8, the animal was found down, apparently in a fit. He was able to get up, however, without assistance. He frothed at the mouth and was weak in the hind legs, but was able to run about. When down he kicked about convulsively. At 10.20 his pulse was 80 and fairly strong. At 10.25 he had apparently recovered and showed no further marked symptoms. He had eaten very little of the material fed, and the poisoning apparently resulted from the feeding of the preceding day.

On the morning of September 9 the uneaten material was removed and at noon he was given 4 pounds of fresh-ground Cicuta roots with a half pound of cut hay.

At 5.55 p. m. he was found down on his left side, kicking convulsively and unable to rise. When raised to his feet, however, he walked to the side of the corral. Respiration was 28 and rather deep. He was fairly strong and able to run about the corral rather actively, so it was difficult to take his pulse. From the time he was found down and helped up he showed no marked symptoms except weakness and uncertain movements of his head. He appeared abnormally excitable, starting at the slightest sound or movement, sometimes giving a sudden start without apparent cause. At 6.55 p. m. he was found down again. He was lying on his belly and unable to rise. His temperature was 102.5°; pulse, 128. At 6.56 he had a convulsion with opisthotonos, followed by violent kicking of the fore and hind legs, rolling over on his side. At 6.58 he managed to rise; his pulse was 132; his head moved about in a spasmodic way, resembling hiccoughs, and suggested spasmodic contractions of the diaphragm. At 7 he was standing with his legs braced apart, unable to walk. His pulse was 172. At 7.06 he fell down again and went into a violent convulsion, more severe than the preceding. His head was drawn up, with his chin against the breast, apparently held by a violent muscular contraction. He then rolled over upon his side with the head thrown back. This was followed by violent movements of his legs and head. Then he lay upon his belly, his legs doubled under him and the hind legs extended. His breathing was labored and the hiccoughing or spasmodic jerking of the sides and head continued. At 7.09 he was still on his belly and unable to rise. His pulse was 180. He was raised to his feet. When his shoulders were raised he fell again, but when his hind quarters were raised he managed to get up, or, in other words, apparently he was especially weak in his hind legs, but was able to use his fore legs. At 7.20 he was able to walk a little when urged. At 8 he was still on his feet and able to walk about, but weak in his hind legs. His pulse was 140 and rather strong. He passed a large quantity of urine. He occasionally belched gas and ground his teeth. The hiccoughing had practically stopped.

From this time on there were no noticeable symptoms, and on the morning of September 10 he was turned back with the band in the pasture. He weighed at the time 86 pounds, showing that during the feeding he had lost 5 pounds. All told, he had eaten 45 pounds of roots. It is to be noted, however, that the feeding was continued over quite a long period and that the poisoning may be considered to have resulted from a comparatively small amount eaten within a short time.

Case No. 125.

Case No. 125 (a wether) was brought in for Cicuta feeding on August 24. This sheep weighed 100 pounds at 6 p. m. on August 25. Feeding was commenced at 10 a. m. on August 26, when it was given leaves, stems, and seeds of Cicuta. This feeding was continued during August 26 and 27. Because of lack of material none was fed on August 28 and 29, but the feeding was resumed on August 30. Because of lack of material no more was fed on August 31 and September 1, but the feeding was resumed on September 2 and continued to September 12.

The animal ate with fair readiness the fresh young leaves and succulent stems, but objected to the dried material, and it was rather difficult to make it clean up the stems and the seed tops. Up to August 30 fresh plants were fed, the seeds being rather green. From September 2 to 6 the material was dry and was eaten less readily. From September 7 to 11 the material was fresher, but the seed tops were past maturity. It is estimated that in the course of the feeding the animal ate 91 pounds. The plant produced no toxic effect and the sheep was turned out on September 12, apparently in good condition. It weighed at this time 94 pounds, having lost 6 pounds in the course of the experiment.

It should be noted that the feeding was rather desultory in character and was extended over such a long time that it could not be considered as a conclusive experiment as to the tops, although the impression among the observers was that the tops were not injurious.

Case No. 102.

Case No. 102 was brought in for feeding with Cicuta on September 14. At 8 p. m., September 15, this wether weighed 93 pounds. At 2.05 p. m., it was fed 1 pound and 9 ounces of ground Cicuta roots. On the morning of September 16 it was given a little hay, mixed with the Cicuta which remained from the feeding of the preceding day. At 5.50 a. m. it was given 1 pound and 10 ounces of ground Cicuta roots and at 9 p. m. was found dead in the corral. It had eaten, all told, in the two days 2 pounds and 8 ounces, or on the basis of 100 pounds of weight $2\frac{7}{10}$ pounds.

This sheep was autopsied on the morning of September 17. It was bloated; there was opisthotonos; it had frothed at the mouth and had evidently kicked about in the corral. It was lying on the left side. The surface of the heart was congested. The left ventricle was contracted and the right ventricle dilated. The lungs were strongly congested, and the inner walls of the trachea and the bronchi inflamed. The walls of the lower part of the ileum and cecum were inflamed. The brain and the membranes of the spinal cord were congested. A piece of the kidney was preserved and sectioned. It showed strong congestion. In the medullary portion the walls of the tubules were in good condition, and the blood was confined to the vessels and was not broken down. In the cortical portion the walls of the tubules were degenerated to some extent. The blood was very abundant and was all through the tissue, not being confined to the vessels. In the cortex a large part of the red corpuscles were "ghosts," the pigment having been broken down and appearing outside the corpuscles in the form of granules. The blood vessels of the tissue of the kidney contained some very large bacteria, probably putrefactive organisms. The conclusion is that this condition of the cortex is due to a combination of an acute nephritis and post-mortem decomposition. A piece of liver was also embedded and sectioned. The liver contained a great deal of blood, most of which was hemolyzed and broken down. The liver cells seemed to be normal. Large numbers of bacteria similar to those found in the kidney were present in the liver.

FEEDING CICUTA TO CATTLE IN 1910.

Case No. 119.

Case No. 119, a heifer weighing 300 pounds, was brought in September 13 for feeding with Cicuta. The animal at that time was in good condition. Feeding was commenced at 8.30 a. m. on September 14, when she was given three roots, to see whether she would eat the plant. At 9.10 a. m. she was fed 1 pound and 5 ounces of the whole roots. At 10.20 a. m. she was found on the ground in a fit. The animal got up, but soon went down again in a violent spasm. She kicked, straightening her legs rapidly, extended her head, and frothed at the mouth, emitting an occasional bellow. She staggered about the corral in a dazed way and went down, kicking violently. An attempt was made to give her a drench of magnesium sulphate and tannin, but her struggles were so violent that it was impossible. A series of photographs taken between 10.27 and 11 show the condition and attitudes assumed. (Pl. IV.) At 10.35 she was given three grains of morphin hypodermically. At 10.45 the struggles were somewhat less violent, perhaps because of exhaustion, and at 10.50 she died.

An autopsy was made immediately. The skin was very much congested, the teats being violet purple in color. The surface of the heart was congested, the left ventricle contracted, and the right expanded, with slight congestion on the inner wall. The lungs and inner walls of the trachea and bronchi were congested. The walls of the anus were inflamed, the kidneys were congested, the brain slightly congested, and the membranes of the spinal cord somewhat congested. The omentum had spots of inflammation 2 or 3 inches across. The lower part of the small intestine was deeply inflamed. The general condition of the circulatory system would indicate that the animal died from respiratory failure. The section of the kidney prepared for microscopic examination showed very great congestion, especially in the cortical portion, where portions of the convoluted tubules appeared somewhat degenerated. The blood vessels and some of the spaces outside the veins were filled with red corpuscles.

Case No. 121.

Case No. 121 was a yearling, weighing about 300 pounds. He was brought in for feeding with Cicuta on the evening of September 8. Feeding was commenced at 9.15 a. m. on September 9, when he received 2½ pounds of whole roots. At noon it was noticed that he was not eating readily. The material had been mixed with cut hay and he had eaten a few of the roots. He was somewhat salivated at this time. Feeding was repeated at 6 p. m. On September 10 he was fed at 10.30 a. m., and at 6 p. m. he was frothing somewhat at the mouth. At this time a large portion of his food had not been eaten. On September 11 he was fed more hay, in order to induce him to clear up the Cicuta; and additional Cicuta was ground and mixed with moist cut hay to induce more complete feeding. This feeding was at 10.15 a. m. At 12 noon he was found salivated, breathing with a peculiar contraction of the nares and elevation of the corners of the mouth.

While the station force was at supper a sound was heard of an animal apparently in distress. This animal was found down on its side, but immediately got up. This was about 7.50 p. m. He walked about uneasily, jerking his head more or less as though having hiccoughs. His pulse was 50 and full. Suddenly he commenced to back, jamming himself first against one side of the corral and then against another, his muscles contracting violently. He went into a fit and fell, the head going down first. He kicked violently and frothed at the mouth. The violent kicking gradually subsided. At 8.05 his pulse was 112 and the breathing was labored and noisy. At 8.08 his pulse was 73 and his respiration 36. At 8.15 the breathing was quieter, the respiration 32.

A little before this he raised himself and lay on his belly with his fore legs doubled under him. Immediately afterwards his eyes were turned in, he struggled convulsively, turned himself about, and fell upon his side, but raised himself again upon his belly. At 8.20 he raised himself again, coming back upon his belly. At 8.22 he had another spasm, going through the same motions. At 8.25 he went into a violent fit. There was marked opisthotonos. He kicked violently, his legs stiffened, standing out rigidly from the body. He frothed at the mouth and was in a strong perspiration.

At 8.30 his pulse was 142. The fit continued, its violence, however, varying. At 8.45 he was given hypodermically a quarter of a grain of strychnin. This was administered in the midst of a fit and he died almost immediately, before the strychnin could have had any effect. Death was caused apparently by respiratory failure, as the action of the heart continued an appreciable time after respiration ceased.

An autopsy was held on September 12. The right auricle was much congested and full of blood. The inner wall of the right ventricle was deeply congested. This ventricle contained little blood and was partly contracted. The left auricle and ventricle contained little blood and were not congested. The wall of the first stomach at the pyloric end was deeply inflamed, as was the wall of the second stomach. On the wall of the fourth stomach were a few inflamed spots. Through the length of the small intestine there were small spots of congestion, while the lower part of the ileum was deeply inflamed. The rectum was somewhat inflamed. The kidneys were congested. The brain was congested, as well as the membranes of the spinal cord. Microscopical section of the kidney showed great congestion, especially in the cortical portion. Portions of the walls of the tubules were degenerated. A great many of the blood corpuscles were broken and stained only very lightly, while through the whole section were granules which did not stain and were probably broken-down blood pigment. The blood vessels also contained bacteria. This animal ate, all told, approximately 10½ pounds, or, on the basis of 1,000 pounds of weight, 35 pounds of Cicuta.

Table II gives a summarized statement of these feeding experiments.

TABLE II.—*Summary of feeding experiments with Cicuta occidentalis, 1910. (Cattle.)*

Animal.	Weight.	Amount fed.	Date or period of feeding.	Part of plant fed.
	Pounds.	*Pounds.*		
No. 119	300	1.5	Sept. 14	Roots.
No. 121	300	10.5 (?)	Sept. 9 to 11	Do.

Animal.	Remedy used.	Result.	Ratio of plant fed to weight of animal.	Amount fed to 1,000 pounds of weight of animal.	Location from which plant fed was obtained.
				Pounds.	
No. 119	None	Death	1 : 200	5	Allison.
No. 121	do	do	1 : 28.5	35	Do.

EXPERIMENTAL WORK OF 1911.

The feeding experiments of 1911 were made to determine whether the tops and seeds of Cicuta are poisonous.

Table III gives a summarized statement of the cattle experiments, the details of which follow.

TABLE III.—*Summary of feeding experiments with Cicuta occidentalis, 1911. (Cattle.)*

Animal.	Weight of animal.	Amount fed.	Period of feeding.	Part of plant fed.
	Pounds.	*Pounds.*		
No. 641	450	76.5	July 26 to 28	Leaves, stems, and flowers, with chopped hay.
No. 648	500	133	July 30 to Aug. 2	Leaves, stems, flowers, and some seed.

Animal.	Period of sickness (until able to stand).	Remedy used.	Result.	Amount fed to 1,000 pounds of weight of animal.	Location from which plant fed was obtained.
				Pounds.	
No. 641	None	None	None	170	Near Castleton.
No. 648	do	do	do	266	Do.

Two head of cattle, Nos. 641 and 648, were fed. No. 641 during the three days from July 26 to 28 received, per 1,000 pounds of weight, 170 pounds of leaves, stems, and flowers of Cicuta. This was fed with a little hay in order to induce the animal to eat it more readily. No. 648 during the four days from July 30 to August 2 received 266 pounds of leaves, stems, flowers, and some seed of Cicuta. Neither of these animals suffered any ill effects from the feeding.

The more extended feeding of the summer was done in the case of sheep. Table IV shows a summary of these experiments. In addition to the thirteen animals listed in the summary, two (Nos. 145 and 152) were brought in for feeding, but ate so little that they are not included in the sum total of the summer's work. Five of the sheep (Nos. 136, 137, 149, 151, and 158) were fed upon the leaves and stems of Cicuta and received, per 100 pounds of weight, from 11.4 pounds, in the case of No. 137, to 143.3 pounds, in the case of No. 158. These amounts were fed in periods varying from one week to about ten days. None of the animals suffered any ill effects from the feeding, although in the case of No. 158 it ate of the plant nearly 50 per cent more than its weight. In all of these cases the sheep were fed exclusively upon the leaves and stems, with the exception of one or two cases, like No. 136, where a little hay was mixed with the material in order to induce the animal to eat it more readily. Nos. 157 and 143 were given leaves, stems, and flowers, mixed with enough hay to induce them to eat it more readily. No. 143 in eleven days ate 16.5 pounds per 100 pounds of weight, while No. 157 in ten days ate 109.1 pounds, or just about the equivalent of its weight. Neither of these animals suffered any ill effects.

TABLE IV.—*Summary of feeding experiments with Cicuta occidentalis, 1911. (Sheep.)*

Animal.	Weight.		Amount fed.	Date or period of feeding.	Part of plant fed.
	Before.	After.			
	Pounds.	*Pounds.*	*Pounds.*		
No. 136	153		19.5	June 17 to 22	Leaves and stems.
No. 137	153		17.5	do	Do.
No. 149	[1] 100		52	June 24 to 30	Do.
No. 151	122		50	do	Do.
No. 157	109½		119.5	July 8 to 18	Leaves, stems, and flowers.
No. 143	122½	120	20.25	July 8 to 19	Stems and flowers.
No. 158	101½		145.5	July 9 to 19	Leaves and stems.
No. 144	103	98	54.5	August 5 to 12	Young seed and seed stems.
No. 135	136	127	2.2	August 16 to 17	Young seed.
No. 142	117	100	2.65	August 19	Seed.
No. 148	137	130	11.5	August 19 to 23	Young seed and seed stems.
No. 151	122		4.4	August 26	Seed.
No. 140	115	106	4.4	August 30	Do.

Animal.	Period of sickness (until able to stand).	Remedy used.	Result.	Amount fed to 100 pounds of weight of animal.	Location from which plant fed was obtained.
				Pounds.	
No. 136	None	None	None	12.7	Near Castleton.
No. 137	do	do	do	11.4	Do.
No. 149	do	do	do	52	Do.
No. 151	do	do	do	41	Do.
No. 157	do	do	do	109.1	Do.
No. 143	do	do	do	16.5	Do.
No. 158	do	do	do	143.3	Do.
No. 144	do	do	do	52.9	Near Hinkle's.
No. 135	do	do	do	1.6	Do.
No. 142	(One spasm?)	do	Recovery	2.3	Do.
No. 148	None	do	None	8.4	Do.
No. 151	do	do	do	3.6	Do.
No. 140	do	do	do	3.8	Do.

[1] Estimated.

Two sheep, Nos. 144 and 148, were fed upon the seeds and seed stems, No. 148 eating 8.4 pounds per 100 pounds of weight and No. 144 receiving 52.9 pounds, or about one-half its own weight. This latter quantity was fed in about a week's time. These animals suffered no harm.

In order to make certain that a large amount of the seeds was taken in a short time, four animals were drenched with the seeds ground up and mixed with enough water to make it possible to administer them in this manner. No. 135 received in two days 1.6 pounds of seed, No. 142 in one day received 2.3 pounds, No. 151 in one day received 3.6 pounds, and No. 140 in one day received 3.8 pounds. Of these animals No. 142 was the only one that sustained any harm.

No. 142 was brought in for feeding on August 18, 1911, weighing at that time 117 pounds. On August 19, at 9.50 a. m., it was given, in a drench with about 1½ quarts of water, 200 grams of ground Cicuta seed. This dose was repeated at 11.15 a. m., 1.50, 3.00, 7.30, and 9.30 p. m. This sheep was given a little hay on August 20, and on August 21, when an attempt was made to turn it out of the corral, it ran part way round the corral, stood, and leaned against the fence, trembling all over. It moved to another part of the corral, and fell there, with the head thrown back, and went into convulsions. These lasted about one minute. The teeth were grated and the muscles contracted. It soon got up, but appeared for several minutes as though dazed. It breathed rapidly for a time and some trembling was noticed for about 15 minutes. The next day, however, it appeared to be all right.

The symptoms were so much like Cicuta poisoning that this condition was considered as due to the effect of the Cicuta seeds, although the poisoning was strangely delayed. None of the animals suffered any harm from the material which they received as a drench.

GENERAL CONCLUSIONS.

SYMPTOMS OF CICUTA POISONING.

Perhaps no better description of Cicuta poisoning has ever been written than that given in 1679 by Wepfer, who tells how children after eating the roots returned home "laeti," one of the little girls tearfully complaining of the selfishness of the others in not giving her her share of the root; he then goes on to tell the symptoms exhibited by each of the children. The following is his description of one case:

Jacobus Maeder, puer sex annorum, capillis albis praeditus, tener vegetus tamen, domum rediit hilaris ac subridens, quasi re bene gesta: paulo post conquerebatur, de praecordiorum dolore & vix verbum effatus, humi prostratus urinam magno impetu ad

Viri altitudinem eminxit: mox terribili aspectu, cum omnium sensuum abolitione convulsus fuit, os arctissime clausit, ut nulla arte aperiri valuerit, dentibus stridebat, oculus mire distorquebat, sanguis ex auribus promanabat: circa praecordia tumidum quoddam Corpus pugni virilis magnitudine, Patris afflicti manum & miserandi Pueri praecordia, maxime circa Cartilaginem ensiformem, validissime feriebat: singultiebat crebro: Vomiturus quandoque videbatur, nihil tamen ore arctissime clauso ejicere valuit: artus mire jactabat & torquebat, saepius caput retrorsum abripiebatur, totumque dorsum incurvabatur in arcum, ut puellus subtus per spatium inter dorsum & stratum inoffense repere potuisset. Cessantibus convulsionibus per momentum matris opem imploravit: mox pari ferocia illis redeuntibus nulla vellicatione, nulla acclamatione, nullove alio ingenio excitari poterat, donec viribus deficientibus expalluit, & manu pectori admota exspiravit. Durarunt haec Symptomata vix ultra horam dimidiam.

Not only is this a vivid and accurate description of the symptoms of Cicuta poisoning, but it has a touch of pathos in the call of the child for assistance from his mother.

Since the time of Wepfer a large number of descriptions of the symptoms of this form of intoxication have been written, most of them being cases of the poisoning of man. There is great uniformity in these descriptions, the difference being mainly in the greater or less stress laid upon particular phases of the symptoms. In minor particulars there has been some contradiction, but this is no more than would be expected, for it is inevitable that among such a large number of observers some would make inaccurate statements.

The symptoms of the lower animals are like those in man, only less marked because of the less susceptible nervous system.

The generally recognized symptoms are as follows:

Pain, especially in the region of the stomach; but it may be quite general in character.

Nausea, leading sometimes to violent vomiting; at others, to spasmodic attempts at vomition without result.

Generally diarrhea and polyuria.

Dilated pupils.

Labored, stertorous breathing, at times irregular.

Sometimes, frothing at the mouth.

Pulse weak, intermittent, and rapid.

Temperature observations have been made in only a few instances, probably due to the fact that most of the recorded cases occurred before the use of the clinical thermometer was common among medical men. According to French, 1866, there is elevation of temperature.

The convulsions are most violent, both tetanic and clonic, accompanied by gnashing of the teeth and trismus, and in violent cases, as in Wepfer's story, by opisthotonos. These convulsions may be accompanied or followed by unconsciousness, and in fatal cases grow more violent until ended by death.

The observation of the cases at Mount Carbon added little to what was already known in regard to the symptoms, but gave a more complete picture.

Excessive salivation, "frothing at the mouth," was generally the first symptom noted, and this occurred in the mild cases. It was followed or accompanied by uneasiness and pain. The animal soon fell in a violent convulsion. Peculiar spasmodic contractions of the diaphragm occurred before and after falling. The convulsions were most violent. The animal would kick, sometimes extending the legs rigidly. It would throw back the head, sometimes with marked opisthotonos, and would bellow and groan as though in great pain. The pupils were dilated and the eyes sometimes turned in or down.

The pulse was weak and rapid, running as high as 180, and respiration was noticed as high as 62.

Gnashing of the teeth and convulsive closing of the jaws were noticed in the Mount Carbon cases.

The convulsions were intermittent and increased in violence in the fatal cases.

In those that recovered there was a gradual slowing of the pulse and respiration.

So far as the observations went there was no change in temperature.

This train of symptoms is so pronounced and so different from those produced by any other poisonous plant in the temperate regions that a diagnosis of Cicuta poisoning is positive and easily made.

AUTOPSY FINDINGS.

A considerable number of autopsies upon man and the lower animals have been reported. Nearly all reports agree as to finding a hyperemia of the brain and central nervous system. Several found inflammation of the walls of the stomach and a fluid condition of the blood. This lack of coagulation of the blood was reported by Wepfer, 1687, and has been noticed repeatedly since that time. Trojanowsky, 1874, says that the poison is antiseptic, as evidenced by the delayed process of decay.

Velten, 1839, found inflammation of the larynx, trachea, and bronchial tubes, and French, 1897, and Nevermann, 1912, reported congested lungs.

Some writers have reported more or less inflammation of the mucous membrane of the stomach.

Three autopsies were made at Mount Carbon—two upon cattle and one upon a sheep. These autopsies confirmed the reports of previous observers, and some additional facts were noted. The left ventricle was contracted and the right dilated, while the walls of the heart were more or less congested. The most marked feature was the extreme congestion of the venous blood vessels. The lungs, kidneys, and membranes of the central nervous system showed strong congestion. The mucous membrane of the trachea and bronchi was inflamed, as were also the inner walls of the small intestine and stomach and in some cases other parts of the alimentary canal.

In the kidneys the congestion was most marked in the cortex and was accompanied with some nephritis. It was noticed that the red blood corpuscles in the kidneys were more or less broken down. Death resulted from respiratory failure.

TOXIC DOSE.

Very little has been known in regard to the toxic dose of Cicuta beyond the fact that only a small quantity is necessary to produce poisonous effects.

Stockbridge, 1814, says that in a fatal case about 1 dram was eaten. Hedrick, 1897, states that a piece the size of a walnut was found by experiment to be sufficient to kill a cow. Other similar estimates have been made, all more or less indefinite. In cases of accidental poisoning it is very difficult to estimate how much has been eaten, and there has been little exact experimental work. About all that has been known is that the rootstock is extremely poisonous and that fatal results have followed the eating of very small quantities.

The experimental work at Mount Carbon gave very little definite information in regard to the toxic dose. The sheep that died ate in two days 2.7 pounds per hundred pounds of weight. From the records, two other sheep which became sick apparently ate a very large quantity of the roots, but the circumstances of the feeding indicate that the actual poisoning was produced by a comparatively small quantity. Heifer No. 119 died as the result of eating 5 pounds per 1,000 pounds of weight in a single day. These deaths occurred at a time when, as stated elsewhere, there is reason to think that the Cicuta is not as poisonous as at other seasons.

All that can be said definitely is that a very small quantity of the root of Cicuta may produce death, but the amount varies with the season and also with the period of time during which it is eaten.

ANIMALS POISONED BY CICUTA.

It is probable that most, if not all, of the higher animals may be poisoned by Cicuta.

Wepfer, 1679, showed experimentally that dogs, wolves, and birds could be poisoned.

Gadd, 1774, says that horses, oxen, cows, and goats are poisoned.

Krause, 1837, describes a case of poisoning of horses and gave details of some experimental work which seemed to corroborate the correctness of his diagnosis.

Oeltze, 1837, and Scholler, 1853, give specific instances of the poisoning of swine.

It has been repeatedly stated in literature that sheep and goats are not affected; where this statement originated is not clear.

Bulliard, 1784, page 99, says that goats eat Cicuta without harm. Gray, 1821, page 508, says that it is poisonous to mankind and kine, but not to horses, sheep, or goats.

Rafinesque, 1828, page 109, states that "sheep and goats eat them [Cicuta plants] with impunity, and even cattle do not appear injured by them when mixed with hay."

Kunkel, 1901, page 935, says that goats and swine are not poisoned, but that horses and all carnivorous animals are very susceptible.

Instances of the poisoning of swine are so specific and given in such detail that we can hardly question their accuracy.

Chesnut, 1901, and Chesnut and Wilcox, 1901, tell of cases of poisoning of sheep in Montana, and the experimental work of the Mount Carbon Station, already detailed, gives conclusive evidence that sheep are affected by Cicuta.

In regard to goats there appears to be no record of definite cases. It does not seem very probable, however, that these animals are immune to Cicuta poisoning.

It will appear later in this paper that Cicuta tops are not poisonous or do not possess enough of the poisonous principle to affect cattle and sheep, and it seems possible that the stories of the immunity of goats may have arisen from cases in which the tops only were eaten and no harmful results followed.

WATER POISONED BY CICUTA ROOTS.

Gadd, 1774, related in some detail a case of poisoning of cattle from drinking water in which were Cicuta roots. Since that time a number of authors have made the statement that cattle trampling the roots along bodies of water from which they drink have rendered the water poisonous. While this may be possible, the evidence does not seem very conclusive.

THE PART OF THE PLANT WHICH IS POISONOUS.

There seems to have been some difference of opinion as to whether or not the whole plant of Cicuta is poisonous. There is a general consensus in regard to the toxic properties of the root, but authorities are contradictory in their statements about the stems and leaves.

Gadd, 1774, states that the poison is mostly in the root and lower leaves.

Rafinesque, 1828, page 109, says that "even cattle do not appear injured by them [the stems and leaves] when mixed with hay."

Schünemann, 1891, says "die ganze Pflanze ist sehr giftig."

Krause, 1837, gives the details of the supposed poisoning of horses by Cicuta in hay. He fed the stems and leaves experimentally to three horses. All became sick and two died.

Hedrick, 1897, says "it is probable that the poisonous constituent is found only in the underground stem and the roots."

Ladd, 1899, states that the roots and seeds are especially poisonous and that the tops are poisonous in hay.

Brodie, 1901, experimenting with *Cicuta vagans*, fed all parts of the plant in May, July, and August without results, but killed an animal in November after the stems and leaves were dead.

Chesnut and Wilcox, 1901, page 82, speaking of *Cicuta occidentalis*, say:

> Field observations indicate that leaves and stems, including the basal portion of this plant, at least during the early stages of growth, contained sufficient poison to produce death. The roots contain a virulent poison.

Blankinship, 1903, page 89, states that the roots and foliage are more poisonous in early spring and that cases are reported of poisoning from eating "slough hay." It is to be presumed that these latter cases were poisoned by the tops.

It appears, therefore, that the preponderance of opinion, we can hardly say evidence, is in favor of the whole plant being poisonous. This subject is discussed in the experimental part of this paper (pp. 15–17).

The feeding experiments at Mount Carbon show that there is little danger, if any, from the aerial parts of the plant. In 1911, Cicuta tops, from the time they were 8 inches to a foot in height until maturity, were fed to sheep with no ill effects. The quantity fed was many times that which would be taken in grazing. It is possible that just as the plants are starting to grow the shoots may be harmful, but it seems more probable that at times the animals poisoned get some of the rootstock. In the experimental work with seeds the animals were drenched with 1.6 to 3.8 pounds of seed to 100 pounds of their weight and only one animal showed symptoms of poisoning. This quantity of seed is evidently vastly more than a sheep could obtain in hay.

It seems clear, then, that hay containing Cicuta tops and seeds is harmless, and that practically the only danger from the plant is from ingestion of the roots.

SEASON WHEN CICUTA IS MOST POISONOUS.

It is generally stated that the plant is most poisonous in the spring. Some authors say that as the stored material of the rootstock is used up in the growth of the plant, it ceases to be poisonous. Certainly most cases of poisoning occur in the spring.

Hedrick, 1897, pages 7 to 9, gives notes of experiments of Prof. French in feeding roots of *Cicuta vagans* in March. One 2-year-old heifer died in an hour and a half from eating not more than 2 drams of one root. Another one was fed "two bulbs the size of an egg" and died in two hours and a half. The bulbs were kept growing in a greenhouse, and feeding experiments conducted early in May, in which several times the quantity used in March produced no ill effects. This seemed to prove conclusively that the roots diminish in toxicity as the growth progresses.

The experimental work at Mount Carbon gave very little exact information in regard to this. The feeding of roots occurred from the middle of August until September 21. Of the sheep, two were made sick and one died. The two cattle experimented upon died. In all cases the quantity eaten was considerably more than that reported by others as poisonous in the spring. The smallest quantity was in the case of No. 119, which ate five pounds per 1,000 pounds of weight, September 14. Of course, at this season, the middle of September, the plant is mature, and if the toxic principle accumulates in the rootstock it might be expected to be as poisonous as in the spring unless some chemical change takes place during the winter. The experiments in August indicate that the roots are poisonous at that time. It seems probable that they are poisonous at all times of the year, but that the toxicity is very much diminished during the growing season of the plant.

REMEDIES FOR CICUTA POISONING.

It was noticed by the older authors that when the eating of Cicuta was followed by vomiting, the patient usually recovered. The logical remedy, then, is an emetic, and when this is given promptly with the first symptoms the prognosis is favorable. What is known of the poisonous principle, cicutoxin, would indicate that it is probably dissolved in the stomach slowly and with some difficulty, and that prompt evacuation of the stomach may remove most of the trouble. The emetic is logically followed by a cathartic to facilitate elimination.

When the convulsions are violent, some form of opium may be given to control them, but the main reliance must be upon the emetic. This has been the treatment used through the whole history of Cicuta poisoning, and no change has been made in modern times beyond the use of more efficient means of emptying the stomach.

In the practical handling of poisoned live stock little can be accomplished in the great majority of cases. The convulsions are so violent that it is difficult to give any remedy *per os*.

Chesnut and Wilcox, 1901, page 85, recommend hypodermic injections of morphin to control the convulsions, giving sheep 1½ grains and cattle and horses 3 to 10 grains. This may assist in bridging over the period of convulsions, and doubtless a purgative would help in carrying off the effects of the poison. Most cases, however, are hopeless, and to reduce the losses attention should be paid to the obvious methods of prevention rather than to any remedies.

SUMMARY.

(1) The poisonous properties of Cicuta have been recognized since the middle of the seventeenth century, and a large number of cases of poisoning of men and animals have been reported.

The toxic principle has been separated and its properties determined. This toxic principle is probably common to all species and there is reason to think that all species are equally poisonous.

(2) There is a definite train of symptoms, marked by nausea, pain, and violent convulsions, which makes it easy to diagnose cases of Cicuta poisoning.

The prominent lesions, as found in autopsies, are congestion of the lungs, kidneys, and central nervous system, with inflammation of the alimentary canal.

(3) So far as known, all the higher animals are poisoned by Cicuta.

(4) The quantity necessary to poison is very variable, depending probably on the stage of growth. The plant is very poisonous at all times.

(5) The toxic principle is largely confined to the rootstock. The tops under ordinary circumstances are not poisonous, and neither the tops nor the seeds when found in hay are a source of danger.

(6) The best remedy is an emetic. Very little can be done for poisoned live stock.

LITERATURE CITED.

The following bibliography includes only the titles of articles cited in this paper. A full bibliography of Cicuta has been prepared and is filed for reference in the Office of Poisonous Plants.

Bigelow, Jacob.
1817. American Medical Botany, v. 1, Boston, p. 125–132, pl. 12.

Blankinship, J. W.
1903. The loco and some other poisonous plants in Montana. Montana Agricultural Experiment Station, Bulletin 45, p. 89–91, fig. 3.

Boehm, R.
1876. Ueber den giftigen Bestandtheil des Wasserschierlings (*Cicuta virosa*) und seine Wirkungen; ein Beitrag zur Kenntniss der Krampfgifte. Archiv für Experimentelle Pathologie und Pharmakologie, Bd. 5, Heft 4/5, p. 279–310.

Brandt, J. F., Phoebus, Philipp, and Ratzeburg, J. T. C.
1838. Abbildung und Beschreibung der in Deutschland Wild Wachsenden und in Gärten im Freien Ausdauernden Giftgewächse nach Natürlichen Familien Erläutert, Abt. 1, Berlin, p. 109–111, pl. 29.

Brodie, D. A.
1901. Poison parsnips in western Washington. Washington Agricultural Experiment Station, Bulletin 45, 12 p., 1 fig.

Bulliard, Pierre.
1784. Histoire des plantes vénéneuses et suspectes de la France. Paris, p. 97–99.

Caillard.
1829. Empoisonnemens par la Ciguë vireuse et par l'émétique; prompte guérison. La Clinique des Hopitaux et de la Ville, t. 4, no. 9, p. 33–34.

Chesnut, V. K.
1901. Some poisonous plants of the northern stock ranges. U. S. Department of Agriculture, Yearbook, 1900, p. 310–314, fig. 39, pl. 33.

——— and Wilcox, E. V.
1901. The stock-poisoning plants of Montana; a preliminary report. U. S. Department of Agriculture, Division of Botany, Bulletin 26, p. 80–86, pl. 7–8.

Dioscorides, Pedanius, of Anazarbos.
[1549]. De Medica Materia, Francofurti, lib. 4, cap. 67; lib. 6, cap. 11; p. 510.

Dragendorff, Georg.
1898. Die Heilpflanzen, Stuttgart, p. 487.

Ely, William, and Muhlenberg, Henry.
1815. Venomous qualities of the water-hemlock, or Cicuta maculata, an indigenous plant of North America. Medical Repository, v. 17 (n. s., v. 2), p. 303–304.

Flora Danica, v. 2 [fasc. 4], Hafniae, pl. 208.
1765.

French, H. T.
1897. Cattle poison. Oregon Agricultural Experiment Station, Press Bulletin, v. 1, no. 5, 1 p.

French, S. P.
1866. Poisoning by hemlock. Boston Medical and Surgical Journal, v. 74, no. 21, p. 428–429.

Gadd, P. A.
1774. Anmärkningar om Cicuta, och upgift at utrota denna giftiga Växt infrån Ängar och Beteshagar. Kongl. Vetenskaps Academiens Handlingar, v. 35, Juli/Aug./Sept., p. 231–244.

For a German translation, see Anmerkungen über die Cicuta und Vorschlag dieses giftige Gewächs von Wiesen und Weiden auszurotten. Der Königl. Schwedischen Akademie der Wissenschaften Abhandlungen, Bd. 36, 1774, p. 236–248. 1781.

Gesner, Konrad.
1541. Historia Plantarum. Paris, 261 p.
1561. Horti Germaniae. *In* Cordus, Valerius. In hoc Volumine Continentur Valerii Cordi Simesusij Annotationes in Pedacij Dioscoridis Anazarbei de Medica Materia Libros V, p. 253.

Gray, Asa.
[1908.] New Manual of Botany. Ed. 7, New York, p. 614, fig. 825.

Gray, S. F.
1821. A Natural Arrangement of British Plants. London, v. 2, p. 507–508, 513–514.

GREENWAY, JAMES.
1793. An account of a poisonous plant, growing spontaneously in the southern part of Virginia. (Extract.) Transactions, American Philosophical Society, v. 3, p. 234–239.

HAZELTINE, RICHARD.
1818. Fatal effects of a poisonous root. New-England Journal of Medicine and Surgery, v. 7 (n. s., v. 2), no. 3, p. 219–222.

HEDRICK, U. P.
1897. A plant that poisons cattle—Cicuta. Oregon Agricultural Experiment Station, Bulletin 46, 12 p., 4 pl.

HELDS, GOTTFRIED, WEINMANN, J. H., and GORITZ, J. A.
1723. Von der Cicuta aquatica, und denen aus Geniessung derselben erfolgten jähen Todesfällen. Sammlung von Natur- und Medicin-Geschichten, 1722, Winter-Quartal, p. 285–294.

KRAUSE.
1837. Ueber die bei Pferden nach dem Genusse von trockenem Wasserschierling (*Cicuta virosa*) beobachtungen Zufälle. Magazin für die Gesammte Thierheilkunde, Jahrg. 3, p. 238–248.

KUNKEL, A. J.
1901. Handbuch der Toxikologie, Hälfte 2, Jena, p. 934–935.

LADD, E. F.
1899. A case of poisoning.—Water hemlock. North Dakota Agricultural Experiment Station, Bulletin 35, p. 307–310, 1 fig.

MALY, JOS.
1844. Über die Vergiftungen mit vegetabilischen Mitteln überhaupt, und mit dem Wasserschierling, *Cicuta virosa*, insbesondere, nebst Andeutung einiger Antidote. Österreichische Medicinische Wochenschrift, Quartal 3, No. 39, p. 1065–1068; No. 40, p. 1097–1100.

NEVERMANN.
1912. Vergiftung durch Wasserschierling. Veröffentlichungen aus den Jahres-Veterinär-Berichten der Beamteten Tierärzte Preussens. Jahrg. 10, 1909, T. 2, p. 39.

OELTZE.
1837. Vergiftungszufällen bei Schweinen. Sanitäts-Bericht für die Provinz Brandenburg, 1835, p. 381–383. Also in Magazin für die Gesammte Thierheilkunde, Jahrg. 7, Quartalheft 2, p. 256–257, 1841, under title Wahrscheinliche Vergiftung mehrerer Schweine durch Wasserschierling.

POHL, JULIUS.
1894. Zur Kenntniss des giftigen Bestandtheils der Oenanthe crocata und der Cicuta virosa. Archiv für Experimentelle Pathologie und Pharmakologie, Bd. 34, Heft 3/4, p. 259–267.

PŘIBRAM, R.
1900. Ein Fall von Vergiftung mit Wasserschierling. Archiv für Kriminal-Anthropologie und Kriminalistik, Bd. 4, Heft 1/2, p. 166–173.

RAFINESQUE, C. S.
1828. Medical Flora, v. 1, Philadelphia, p. 107–110, pl. 22.

RAY, JOHN.
1704. Historia Plantarum, v. 3, Londoni, lib. 8, p. 257.

REGEL, ALBERT.
1876–1877. Beitrag zur Geschichte des Schierlings und Wasserschierlings. Bulletin, Société Impériale des Naturalistes, Moscou, t. 51, pt. 1, no. 1, p. 155–203, 1876; t. 52, pt. 1, no. 1, p. 1–52, 1877.

SCHOEPF, J. D.
1787. Materia Medica Americana Potissimum Regni Vegetabilis, Erlangae, p. 36. See Linné, Carl von, Amœnitates Academicae, v. 10, Erlangae, 1790.

SCHOLLER.
1853. Vergiftung mit Schierling (*Cicuta virosa*). Magazin für die Gesammte Thierheilkunde, Jahrg. 19, Quartalheft 2, p. 262–263.

SCHÜNEMANN, H.
1891. Die Pflanzen-Vergiftungen, Braunschweig, p. 15–17, fig. 2.

SCHWENCKE, M. W.
1756. Verhandeling over de Waare Gedannte, Aart, en Uytwerking', der Cicuta aquatica Gesneri, of Groote-Waterscheerling. 'S Gravenhage. 54 p., 4 pl.
1776. Abhandlung von dem grossen Wasserschierling, desselben Kennzeichen und Wirkungen. Aus dem Holländischen übersetze von A. S. Müller. Munster und Leipzig, 37 p., 3 pl.

SLADE, H. B.
1903. Some conditions of stock poisoning in Idaho. Idaho Agricultural Experiment Station, Bulletin 37, p. 157–190, 3 fig., 2 pl.

STEARNS, FREDERICK.
1858. The medicinal plants of Michigan. Proceedings, American Pharmaceutical Association, 7th annual meeting, p. 253.

STOCKBRIDGE, JOHN.
1814. Account of the effects produced by eating a poisonous plant, called Cicuta maculata. New England Journal of Medicine and Surgery, v. 3, no. 4, p. 334–337.

TROJANOWSKY, C.
1874. Zur Wasserschierlingwurzel-Vergiftung. Dorpater Medicinische Zeitschrift, Bd. 5, Heft 3, p. 181–229.

TRUMEL, J. A.
1838. Quels sont les caractères des diverses plantes connues sous le nom de Ciguë? Les comparer entre elles, et indiquer leurs propriétés médicales. Thèses Faculté de Médicine de Paris, No. 239, p. 5–9.

VELTEN.
1839. Vergiftung durch Cicuta virosa. General-Bericht, Königl. Rheinisches Medicinal-Collegii, [Koblenz], 1837, p. 183–186. Also in Wochenschrift für die Gesammte Heilkunde, No. 19, p. 308–311, 1840.

WEPFER, J. J.
1679. Cicutae Aquaticae Historia et Noxae. Basiliae, 336 p., 5 fig.
1687. Cicutae aquaticae noxa. Miscellanea Curiosa sive Ephemeridum Medico-Physicarum Germanicarum Academiae Imperialis Leopoldinae Naturae Curiosorum, [Norimbergae], dec. 2, ann. 6, p. 221–241.
For a German translation, see Von der Schädlichkeit des Wasserschierlings. Der Römisch-Kaiserlichen Akademie der Naturforscher Auserlesene Medicinisch-Chirurgisch-Anatomisch-Chymisch- und Botanische Abhandlungen, [Nürnberg], t. 16, p. 203–224, 1767.
For a French abstract, see Sur les mauvais effets de la Ciguë aquatique. Collection Académique, [Dijon et Paris], t. 7, p. 451–454, 1766.

WIKSZEMSKI, ADAM.
1875. Beiträge zur Kenntniss der Giftigen Wirkung des Wasserschierlings (*Cicuta virosa*). Dorpat, 58 p. Inaugural-Dissertation.

WOOD, G. B., and BACHE, FRANKLIN.
[1907.] The Dispensatory of the United States of America. Ed. 19, rev., Philadelphia, p. 1449.

O

WASHINGTON : GOVERNMENT PRINTING OFFICE : 1914

Spotted something that isn't quite right?

Let us know and we'll fix it for future reprints. And as a thank you for your diligence, we'll send you a free Sothis book of your choice.

publisher@sothis.press

This page intentionally left blank

Made in United States
Cleveland, OH
06 November 2026

47793877R00023